Simple Healthy Smoothies For The 5:2 Diet

Emily Hanson

ISBN:
ISBN-13: 978-1484941706

To Donna

For all her kindness and
encouragement

CONTENTS

Page

Introduction

As a child I was teased mercilessly in the playground about my size. I wasn't exactly fat, just 'podgy' but the unkind remarks hurt. As a teenager I became increasingly conscious of my weight, especially as my brother and sister were both much slimmer than me. My self-esteem plummeted even lower and I developed a very poor body image.

As an adult I was lucky to marry someone who loved me for myself (and still does). However, because of my low self-esteem I became depressed and turned to eating for comfort. I soon billowed out and by the time I was thirty-five I weighed an unhealthy eighteen stone, completely unacceptable for my height of five foot six.

I tried every diet I came across but found it impossible to stick with any of them for very long, despite my determination. My weakness for my favourite foods, especially anything sweet, led to failure each time.

* * *

The 5:2 diet is one of the easiest diets to follow, both in concept and in practice. This simplicity, combined with the unrivalled effectiveness of its method, has fuelled its rapid growth in popularity to make it one of the most used diets today.

When I first heard about this diet, the idea sounded so simple that I was admittedly skeptical. Surely something so straightforward would have been brought to light before now were it effective, instead of all those complicated nutrient-specific regimes I'd been hopelessly working my way through for longer than I cared to remember? Had it not been for the endorsements by some recognised members of the scientific community I may in fact not even have given it a try.

I'm glad I did! Not only did I find the 5:2 diet particularly easy to stick to, it also very quickly proved to be exceptionally effective. I found I actually began to enjoy this new way of eating and was spurred on even more by the fast results that came with it. I lost weight surprisingly fast: in the first couple of months alone I lost 24 pounds. And after six months I'm already halfway towards my target weight of 147 pounds (10 ½ stone), having shed just under four stone. The biggest spinoff, though, has been that my self-esteem has improved immensely. I get up every day feeling better about myself than I ever did. My husband is delighted with my new-found confidence (which is just as well as he's footing the bill for new clothes to fit my slimmer frame!).

Being kind to myself if I am having a bad day, which might be completely unrelated to food, is an effective way to deal with any distress. In the past I often used food to comfort myself but then I discovered rather more healthy ways to make myself feel better. It might be a bit of retail therapy but more often it's something that costs nothing, like going into the garden or walking in the park, listening to the various sounds, feeling the sun warming my skin and looking at the beauty of nature around me. I don't try to push away any feelings inside me – I simply notice them and accept that they are there but am aware of the need to look outward as well.

* * *

For those who are completely new to the 5:2 diet, the method is very easy to understand. For five days of each week there are no rules – no foods to avoid and no calorie counting. You can simply eat or drink as you would normally. Even alcohol is not off-limits!

The other two days, which can be any two days you like, are your low calorie days. On these days you restrict your calories to 500 (or 600 for men). While this does initially require some degree of effort, the knowledge that on the following day you will be able to eat as much as you like should be more than enough to get you through the difficult periods. Furthermore, as your body becomes accustomed to this new way of eating, not only do the low calorie days become easier but you'll likely find yourself wanting less to eat on the other days too.

Further to the weight loss benefits offered by the diet, an increasing amount of research also suggests there are a number of other health advantages to be gained by this way of eating. The 5:2 diet has been shown to reduce cholesterol and improve blood sugar levels and is believed to significantly lessen the risk of serious illnesses such as diabetes, heart disease and cancer, as well as protecting the brain from diseases such as Parkinson's and Alzheimer's.

As there is a certain amount of self-discipline required for the two low calorie days each week, I decided fairly early on to spice these days up by adding as much variety to what I ate and drank as possible. Obviously, the 500 calorie limit does cancel out certain high-calorie foods on your diet days; however, with a bit of creativity and variety these two days can become just as, if not even more, enjoyable.

One of the most effective ways I found to add this variety was by experimenting with different types of smoothies. They are a great way of packing healthy nutrients into a tasty drink, and can also be surprisingly filling. They are perfect for any meal, whether it be to give you the boost you need in the morning, to keep you going throughout the day or to help you relax in the evening.

Having always previously thought of smoothies as fruit-based drinks, I was pleasantly surprised to discover that actually there are many other foods that work just as well. In fact, something that became very quickly apparent was that often it was the really unexpected combinations that ended up with the most delicious drinks, as you will find in some of the recipes that follow.

The most common question people ask when it comes to making smoothies is whether you will need a juicer. This is really down to personal choice. You may wish to juice harder fruits and vegetables, such as apples and carrots; however, for simplicity, I use pre-packaged juice from the supermarket. However, I prefer juices not made from concentrates as the process they go through in the making destroys or diminishes many nutrients. So I look for ones that are labelled "not from concentrate" or "freshly squeezed".

You will, however, need a blender (I've tried using the lawnmower instead and it's far too messy!). If you are really serious about making smoothies, it's worth investing in a good quality one (blender, that is, not lawnmower), with a large, easy-to-clean jug, a heavy base to keep it steady when in use and a multi-speed motor. The highest speed will be necessary for crushing ice and breaking down hard foods such as celery and carrot. If it is equipped with a pulse control, so much the better: among other things, this feature helps to dislodge any lumps of food that may get stuck beneath the blades, as well as giving you an extra degree of control over the whole process of preparing a smoothie. This is not the place to get into technicalities but if you don't already own a blender I would recommend doing a bit of research online before buying one: there are plenty of websites with helpful guidance and it's worth noting that it's not always the most expensive ones that do the best job!

A citrus squeezer also comes in handy for your oranges, lemons and limes.

All the recipes in this book are designed for a single serving. Obviously, if you wish to make any more than this you can simply scale the amounts up accordingly. I have also listed calorie counts for each recipe in order to help you pick the smoothie that fits in best with any other meal/s you may have planned for the day.

Over time I have developed a passion for smoothie

making and in this book I have shared with you some of my favourites. I've tried my hardest to be as accurate as possible with measurements based on the ones I have used. However, the great thing is that there is no exact science when it comes to making smoothies and therefore do feel free to adjust any of the amounts listed according to taste (making sure to also take into account any differences in calories if you do this!).

In case you are puzzled by the use of the words "blend", "whizz" and "blitz" in the recipe instructions and wonder what the difference is between them, I ought to explain that there is no difference at all. Having started by using the word "blend" repeatedly I thought maybe the reader would prefer a bit of variety (and it made it more interesting for me, too!).

Although the 5:2 diet is safe for most people, it is not something to be undertaken by pregnant women, people with a history of eating disorders or children. If you have any type on ongoing medical condition or any health problems at all, you need to consult your GP before embarking on any diet.

One more point that needs to be made is that, although I have done my best to ensure that all the details within these pages are as accurate as possible, I apologise if anything has been printed incorrectly or is misunderstood. I am, after all, only human!

Practically Speaking

In order to help you get the most out of this book, I'm taking the liberty of adding a few practical hints. I hope you'll forgive me if some of them seem obvious but in my experience it's often the obvious that gets overlooked.

It should, for instance, go without saying that having everything you need at the ready before you start on a recipe can make life much easier and get things done faster and more tidily. But sadly, not all of us are as well organised as we should be (the voice of personal experience again!), so it's worth mentioning a basic list of items that you will need for most of the recipes and that could be kept together for ease of finding them when you need them.

The main one (and because of its size, the hardest to mislay) is your aforementioned blender. Also on your list will be a sharp knife, a measuring jug and a small measuring glass (or even a medicine pot) for measuring out smaller amounts of liquid. And don't forget the citrus squeezer. A teaspoon and a tablespoon are important items or, better still, a set of measuring spoons actually made for the purpose: I have a set that measures out one tablespoon, one teaspoon, half a teaspoon and a quarter of a teaspoon. You'll still need a proper spoon for scooping out the insides of some fruit such as papaya and kiwi.

As I said earlier, there are no fixed rules to smoothie-making; but calorie-counting is an important part of this book and it's helpful in this respect to be able to measure accurately (though not obsessively!).

Although some people may prefer to use a juicer to extract the juice from hard fruit and vegetables, being someone who hates having to clean two appliances when one will do, I have found that there are ways round this (some of us will go to no end of trouble to find the easy way to do something!). One is to chop anything hard into very small chunks to make sure the blades can process them. To this end I bought a very useful gadget of the type often seen demonstrated on TV shopping channels: a multi-purpose device with a variety of blades set into the lid of a plastic box and which does everything from grating and slicing to chopping potatoes into the right size for making French fries . It's ideal for making small carrot batons and for chopping firm apples into little bits. The only downside to this wonderful device is the potential to slice fingers as well, as I found out when I first bought it. So if you buy one, please handle it more carefully than I did!

The other way to process fruit like apples and pears is to use them only when they are very ripe and soft. Pears in particular produce lovely juice when they are soft, whereas for eating purposes you'd probably prefer them firmer.

In the recipes that follow, I haven't mentioned the repetitive tasks such as washing all fruit and vegetables, taking the stones out of peaches or peeling bananas. That would be patronising!

Of course, your main reason for reading this book is, I'm sure, to be able use smoothies as part of your 5:2 low-calorie days. To make this as easy as possible I have arranged all the recipes in ascending order of calorie values (i.e. lowest first). Each smoothie has its calorie count clearly displayed after the list of ingredients. They range from a miserly 65 calories up to a hefty 246 calories (nearly half your daily allowance). The idea is that you can use these smoothies to fit in with the way you intend to follow the diet. For instance, many prefer to have two meals rather than three on these days. In that case, having decided what to eat for your main meal, and having worked out the calorie content, you could then select a smoothie for your other meal that would make up the rest (or nearly the rest) of your allowance. If you have planned three meals for each low-calorie day, you could do the same, adding the values of the two other meals together and supplementing them with a smoothie to make up the shortfall.

Because tastes differ, I've tried to cater for as wide a range as possible, from very sweet to spicy and savoury. And to make it even easier for you to experiment without losing track of the calories, I've followed the recipes with a chart that lists every ingredient used together with its calorie content in standard measurements, so that you can "mix and match" armed with facts and figures.

When I started making smoothies, I kept visiting the market or supermarket for fresh fruit on an almost daily basis. But having gone through the messy job of slicing up a mango and wondering whether I didn't have anything better to do with my time, I started buying frozen fruit. This has pretty much the same calorie count, tastes just as good, is easier to control the amounts you want, saves adding ice and leaves much less mess to clear up. Fresh and frozen fruit are for practical purposes interchangeable as far as smoothies are concerned. But if mango-slicing is your thing, don't let me stop you!

Sometimes I freeze freshly-bought fruit such as bananas and oranges to use in smoothies at a later date.   The skin of a banana turns black on freezing but this in no way impairs the flesh, which becomes very creamy on being defrosted (it's best to peel them before they are completely defrosted for ease of handling).   The freezing process seems to make oranges give up their juice more readily after defrosting.   Grapes also freeze well and can be used instead of ice cubes.

Occasionally a recipe calls for half or less of a fruit. What can you do with the rest of it (apart, that is, from cheating and eating it!)? One very good way to use it is to cut it into appropriately sized pieces to use as the basis for a fruit salad the next day.   To avoid banana or apple slices turning brown, sprinkle them with a little lemon juice and refrigerate them.

You'll find several references to stevia in the recipes.   For anyone unfamiliar with this, it's a natural sweetener that has the big advantage for dieters in being calorie-free and has no nasty aftertaste like some of the artificial sweeteners.   It has become increasingly popular in recent years and is readily available in most supermarkets / grocery stores under a number of brand names.

As for almond milk, rice milk and soya milk, I realise that almond, rice and soya are not mammals and that their products are therefore not, technically speaking, milk.   However, milk is the name by which they're generally known so that is how I'll refer to them.

If you find a smoothie that sounds good to you but is too high in calories for your needs, try substituting the liquid for something such as for almond milk or coconut water, both of which have a very low calorie content (and of course there's water, which is zero-calorie rated). Or simply use a little less of an ingredient. These measures will, obviously, change the taste but I've found that in smoothie-making, most of the liquids in these recipes combine well with all the fruit and most of the vegetables. And it's fun experimenting!

Although many of these recipes require a tall glass for serving, some produce less liquid, which looks better in a smaller glass. Filling a small glass, instead of having a half empty tall one, has the psychological effect of enjoying a larger drink. It may be an optical illusion but it definitely feels much more satisfying!

Smoothies are often thought of as a "holiday" drink, bought at places such as tropical beach bars, so why not make the most of yours by embellishing it with a little umbrella, a very wide straw and a wedge of orange, lemon or lime? You could also sit outdoors to drink it (though if the weather is up to its usual perverse tricks you may prefer to sit indoors and look at a picture of a tropical beach).

I hope you enjoy these smoothies as much as I do and wish you every success eating the 5:2 way. May your dieting go smoothie!

Seventy-Five Smoothie Recipes

Cool Tomato and Cucumber

120ml (4 fl.oz) tomato juice
4 tablespoons fat-free natural yoghurt
112g (4 oz) peeled cucumber
Ice
Mint leaves

65 calories

Pour tomato juice into blender
Spoon in yoghurt
Chop and add cucumber
Add ice
Blend on high setting
Garnish with mint to serve

*Made up mostly of water, cucumbers keep the body
hydrated and help rid our bodies of toxins.
Hydrating the skin around your eyes means fewer
lines and wrinkles in the future so cut off a couple
of thick slices and relax with them over your eyes
for 10 minutes whilst you sip your smoothie*

Cranberry and Ginger

84g (3 oz) cranberries
¼ teaspoon ground ginger
240ml (8fl.oz) coconut water
Stevia to taste
Ice

65 calories

Put cranberries into blender
Add ground ginger
Pour in coconut water
Add stevia as desired
Pop in ice
Blitz thoroughly

Cranberries are rich in vitamin C with very good infection-fighting properties

Fruity Fizz

180ml (6 fl.oz) sparkling water
56g (2 oz) frozen mango slices
56g (2 oz) frozen peach slices
½ apricot, canned
2 mint leaves

66 calories

Pour sparkling water into blender
Carefully add mango and peach slices
Put in apricot
Whizz thoroughly
Garnish with mint before serving

*Peaches are naturally sweet and the Chinese say
that their potassium content prolongs life (but still
take care when crossing the road!)*

Mango, Carrot and Pineapple with Citrus

28g (1 oz) frozen mango chunks
30ml (1 fl.oz) fresh orange juice
30ml (1 fl.oz) carrot juice
30ml (1 fl.oz) pineapple juice
15ml (1 tablespoon) fresh lemon juice
60ml (2 fl.oz) sparkling mineral water
½ teaspoon clear honey

75 calories

Put mango chunks into blender
Pour in the juices and mineral water
Add honey
Blend on a high setting

*The beta-carotene in mango promotes glowing skin
and healthy eyesight*

Watercress with Fruit

14g (½ oz) watercress
42g (1½ oz) pineapple chunks
42g (1½ oz) blueberries
½ small banana
150ml (5 fl.oz) water

87 calories

Put watercress into blender.
Add all the fruit
Pour in water
Combine thoroughly in blender

Watercress is an excellent source of vitamin K
which helps to strengthen bones

Creamy Rhubarb

120ml (4 fl.oz) natural fat-free yoghurt
2 ripe rhubarb stalks
1 tablespoon orange juice
Stevia to taste
60ml (2 fl.oz) water
Ice cubes

94 calories

Spoon yoghurt into blender
Chop and add rhubarb
Pour in orange juice
Add stevia as desired
Pour in water
Add ice cubes
Whizz on high setting until smooth

*The red colour in rhubarb is due to the antioxidant
in it which helps to prevent disease by giving your
immune system a boost*

Almondberry

120ml (4 fl.oz) of almond milk
4 tablespoons natural fat-free yoghurt
84g (3 oz) frozen mixed berries
½ small carrot

96 calories

Pour milk into blender
Spoon in yoghurt
Add berries
Peel, chop and add carrot
Blend until completely smooth

*Almond milk is low in calories, full of vitamins and
minerals and tastes great*

Fruit Sparkler

56g (2 oz) orange sorbet
56g (2 oz) fresh strawberries
56g (2 oz) canned pineapple chunks
120ml (4 fl.oz) sparkling mineral water

102 calories

Scoop sorbet into blender
Halve strawberries and add to blender
Put in pineapple chunks
Pour in water
Blend until combined

*Pineapple is a good source of fibre but low in
calories, sodium, saturated fats and cholesterol
which makes it an ideal weight loss food*

Melon, Mint and Beetroot

168g (6 oz) fresh watermelon, cubed
240ml (8 fl.oz) almond milk
6 mint leaves
4 beet leaves
A few ice cubes

107 calories

Place watermelon in blender
Pour in almond milk
Add mint, beet leaves and ice
Whizz until smooth

The fibre in beetroot leaves increases the amount of good cholesterol (HDL) in our bodies and so helps to prevent heart disease

Veggie Smoothie

120ml (4 fl.oz) low fat natural yoghurt
½ tablespoon onion
1 small stick of celery
1 medium tomato
½ cucumber
Couple of drops Tabasco Sauce
Salt and Pepper

107 calories

Spoon yoghurt into blender
Chop onion and celery finely and add
Slice and add tomato
Peel, chop and add cucumber
Shake in a couple of drops of Tabasco
according to taste
Add salt and pepper
Blend until everything is combined

An accident happened to my brother Jim
When somebody threw a tomato at him
Tomatoes are juicy and don't hurt the skin
But this one was specially packed in a tin

Fibre Filler

180ml (6 fl.oz) almond milk
½ orange
½ lemon
½ peach
2 spinach leaves
1 carrot

111 calories

Pour almond milk into blender
Peel, chop and deseed lemon and orange and
add
Slice peach and add
Pop in spinach leaves
Peel, slice and add carrot
Whizz until smoothly blended

*Every citrus fruit contains fibre which helps you feel
fuller for longer*

Coffee Perk

120ml (4 fl.oz) skimmed milk
60ml (2 fl.oz) strong brewed coffee
½ teaspoon instant coffee
120ml (4 fl.oz) vanilla yoghurt
¼ teaspoon vanilla essence

112 calories

Pour milk and brewed coffee into blender
Add instant coffee
Put in yoghurt and vanilla essence
Combine in blender

*Coffee contains minerals like magnesium and
chromium which help the body use insulin – the
hormone that controls blood sugar*

Parsley, Cranberry and Blueberry

¼ cucumber
120 ml (4 (fl.oz) cranberry juice
10g ($^1/_3$ oz) parsley
84g (3oz) blueberries
Stevia to taste (if you have a sweet tooth)
Ice

117 calories

Peel, chop and put cucumber into blender
Pour in cranberry juice
Chop and add parsley
Blend well
Add blueberries, ice and stevia if desired
Blend again until completely combined

*Parsley contains lots of vitamin K which is
important for prevention of cardiovascular disease
and strokes*

Blueberry-Banana Soya Heaven

240ml (8 fl.oz) soya milk
56g (2 oz) frozen blueberries
½ banana
½ teaspoon vanilla essence
Stevia to taste

117 calories

Pour soya into blender
Add blueberries
Slice and add banana
Put in vanilla essence and add stevia to taste
Whizz until blended

Not just one, but two, superfoods – blueberries and bananas- in this!

Vanilla, Celery and Blueberry Fix

180ml (6 fl.oz) vanilla soya milk
1 celery stalk
84g (3 oz) blueberries
Stevia
Ice

120 calories

Pour soya into blender
Chop celery and place in blender
Add blueberries and ice
Blitz completely

*As well as lowering blood pressure, celery has
cancer preventing properties*

Banana and Strawberry Kiss

2 tablespoons fat-free natural yoghurt
1 small banana
56g (2oz) frozen strawberries
150ml (5 fl.oz) almond milk
Stevia to taste

121 calories

Spoon yoghurt into blender
Slice and add in the banana
Add the strawberries
Pour in almond milk
Blend at the highest speed setting

*Banana thickens and strawberries colour this
creamy smoothie*

Spicy Surprise

56g (2 oz) frozen blueberries
1 teaspoon cocoa powder
1 very small banana
14g (½ oz) baby spinach
Small pinch cayenne pepper
1 teaspoon honey
240ml (8 fl.oz) water

121 calories

Put blueberries into blender
Add cocoa powder
Chop and add banana
Put in spinach
Sprinkle on pepper
Add honey
Pour in water
Blitz until smooth

The flavonoids in cocoa increase the flow of blood and oxygen to the brain

Strawberry Crush

120ml (4 fl.oz) fat-free natural yoghurt
60ml (2 fl.oz) skimmed milk
112g (4oz) strawberries, fresh or frozen

122 calories

Put yoghurt into blender
Pour in milk
Add strawberries
Whizz thoroughly

Some say strawberries can prevent wrinkles; I say,
whether it's true or not they taste delicious!

Peachberry Quencher

60ml (2fl.oz) apple juice
4 tablespoons fat-free vanilla yogurt
84ml (3 oz) frozen peach slices
56g (2 oz) frozen raspberries
180ml (6 fl.oz) water

125 calories

Pour apple juice into blender
Spoon in yoghurt
Add frozen peach slices
Add raspberries
Pour in water
Blend completely

Unsurprisingly, yoghurt is high up in the list of foods that are good for your health – it contains intestine-friendly bacterial cultures that keep your colon healthy.

Melony Green Tea Drink

227g (8 oz) honeydew melon
1 kiwi fruit
120ml (4 fl.oz) water
2 tsp. chopped fresh mint
½ tsp. matcha
Stevia to taste

127 calories

Cut melon into small pieces and place in
blender
Halve kiwi fruit, scoop out flesh and add to
blender
Pour in water
Add mint and matcha
Blend thoroughly
Add stevia to taste

*Matcha green tea is a Japanese tea that comes in
powder form. Studies have shown that drinking
green tea can significantly lower our risk of
developing brain diseases such as Alzheimer's*

Peach and Ginger

120ml (4 fl.oz) rice milk
168g (6 oz) frozen peach slices
¼ teaspoon ground ginger
Ice cubes

128 calories

Pour rice milk into blender
Add peach slices and ginger
Pop in ice cubes
Whizz thoroughly

Rice milk is made from partially milled rice and water and is good for anyone who is lactose intolerant

Sweet Banana Smile

150ml (5 fl.oz) skimmed milk
½ medium banana
2 tablespoons low fat natural yoghurt
1 teaspoon clear honey
¼ teaspoon vanilla essence

128 calories

Pour milk into blender
Slice banana and add to milk
Put in yoghurt
Add honey and vanilla essence
Blend thoroughly

Honey has powerful anti bacterial properties

Banana Spice

1 medium banana
¼ teaspoon ground nutmeg
¼ teaspoon ground cinnamon
¼ teaspoon ground cloves
180ml (6 fl.oz) almond milk
Ice

129 calories

Slice banana and put into blender
Add nutmeg, cinnamon and cloves
Pour in almond milk
Add ice
Blitz until smooth

*Nutmeg is purported to be a brain stimulant,
cinnamon to regulate blood sugar and cloves
contain healthy antioxidants*

Sunny Shake

1 small tomato
56g (2 oz) pineapple pieces
112g (4 oz) frozen mango
120ml (4 fl.oz) almond milk

132 calories

Halve tomato and place in blender
Add pineapple
Put in mango
Pour in almond milk
Blend thoroughly

Tomatoes are high in lycopene which is said to be a good preventative for cancer

Smooth Citrus and Strawberry

120ml (4 fl.oz) fat-free vanilla yogurt
60ml (2 fl.oz) cup orange juice
112g (4 oz) strawberries
2 teaspoons lemon juice
¼ teaspoons lemon zest
Crushed ice

132 calories

Spoon yoghurt into blender
Pour in orange juice
Halve and add strawberries
Add lemon juice and zest
Blend until smooth
Pour over crushed ice and stir

Citrus fruits are high in both vitamin C and fibre

Greenie & Creamie

28g (1 oz) pre-packed baby spinach
168g (6 oz) seedless green grapes
60ml (2 fl.oz) coconut water
Ice as desired

139 calories

Put spinach and grapes into blender
Pour in coconut water
Add ice as desired
Blend until totally smooth

*Coconut water is the liquid found inside a coconut.
It is rich in potassium, which helps the body to
absorb water and also to maintain normal blood
pressure*

Berry Smooth Banana and Broccoli

5 tablespoons natural yoghurt
70g (2½ oz) frozen mixed berries
28g (1 oz) broccoli
60ml (2 fl.oz) skimmed milk
1 small banana

142 calories

Spoon yoghurt into blender
Add mixed berries
Put in broccoli
Pour in milk
Slice and add banana
Blend until completely smooth

Broccoli contains vitamin A, which is essential for healthy eyesight

Cherrynilla

4 tablespoons fat-free vanilla yoghurt
112g (4 oz) of frozen cherries
120ml (4 fl.oz) cranberry juice

144 calories

Spoon yoghurt into blender
Add cherries
Pour in cranberry juice
Whizz until smooth

*Cherries reduce inflammation, are a natural
painkiller and improve the quality of your sleep –
but best without the stones which can damage your
teeth and mess up your blender!*

Cinnamon Spiced Berries

56g (2 oz) blackberries
56g (2 oz) strawberries
56g (2 oz) blueberries
120ml (4 fl.oz) soya milk
Pinch ground cinnamon
Stevia to taste
Ice cubes

149 calories

Cut strawberries in half
Put all berries into blender
Pour in soya milk
Add cinnamon, stevia and ice cubes
Blend until smooth

It is said that cinnamon can boost memory. It certainly has a memorable smell

Carribean Sunset

1 small papaya
1 peach
1 passion fruit
180ml (6fl oz) coconut water
Crushed ice

149 calories

Peel and deseed papaya and put flesh into
blender
Slice and add peach
Slice open passion fruit and scoop flesh with
seeds into blender
Pour in coconut water
Blend thoroughly, pour over crushed ice and
serve

*The seeds in passion fruit are good for you as they
contain lots of fibre which is important for you
because it keeps your large intestine cleaned out
and keeps you regular (the seeds are crunchy too!)*

Spinach and Melon

75ml (2½ fl.oz) fat-free vanilla yoghurt
56g (2 oz) baby spinach leaves
336g (12 oz) honeydew melon
Ice

150 calories

Spoon yoghurt into blender
Tear and add spinach leaves
Chop melon into small chunks and add
Put in a few ice cubes
Whizz until smooth

*Honeydew melons are good for maintaining healthy
skin, hair, and keeping your weight down*

Spiced Carrot, Apple and Orange

120ml (4 fl.oz) carrot juice
½ green apple
1 teaspoons freshly grated ginger
120ml (4 fl.oz) freshly squeezed orange juice
Ice cubes

150 calories

Pour carrot juice into blender
Core, chop and add apple
Add grated ginger
Pour in orange juice
Pop in ice cubes
Blitz until blended

Ginger is a well known cure for nausea and travel sickness; it's antibacterial and excellent for your digestive tract

Quirky Carrot with Apple

120ml (4 fl.oz) carrot juice
60ml (2 fl.oz) apple juice
60ml (2 fl.oz) fat-free natural yoghurt
½ eating apple
¼ teaspoon cinnamon powder
Ice cubes

152 calories

Pour Carrot and apple juices into blender
Spoon in yoghurt
Core, chop and add apple
Sprinkle with cinnamon
Add ice cubes
Blitz until smooth

Apple is good for your skin except when it's thrown at you!

Orange and Yoghurt Paradise

240ml (8 fl.oz) orange juice with bits
4 tablespoons fat-free yoghurt
¼ teaspoon vanilla essence
A few ice cubes

153 calories

Pour orange juice into blender
Spoon in yoghurt
Add vanilla essence and ice cubes
Whizz until blended

Oranges are tangy, sweet and a brilliant source of vitamin C

Funky Melon

1 tablespoon of ground flax seed
60ml (2 fl.oz) skimmed milk
112g (4 oz) watermelon
1 nectarine
Ice

154 calories

Put flax seed into blender
Pour in milk
Deseed watermelon and add flesh to blender
Slice and add nectarine
Add ice and whizz on high setting to blend

*The mildly nutty flavour of the flax seeds goes well
with the fruit and the fibre in it fills you up nicely*

Veggies and Fruits

28g (1 oz) kale leaves without ribs and
stems
120ml (4 fl.oz) apple juice
1 small stalk celery
1 small banana
tablespoon fresh lemon juice
60ml (2fl.oz) water
Ice cubes

156 calories

Shred the kale leaves and put into blender
Pour in apple juice
Chop and add celery and banana
Pour in lemon juice, water and ice cubes
Whizz until smooth

*Kale is a wonderfully healthy vegetable packed with
calcium, soluble fibre, antioxidants and vitamins*

Vital Vitamin Booster

60ml (2 fl.oz) orange juice
56g (2 oz) frozen blackberries
1small kiwi fruit
1 small apricot
60ml (2 fl.oz) prune juice
Ice

158 calories

Pour orange juice into blender
Add blackberries
Halve kiwi fruit, scoop out flesh and put in blender
Chop and add apricot flesh
Pour in prune juice
Add ice
Combine all ingredients on a high setting

All the goodness of vitamins and a small measure of prune juice to keep you regular!

Breezy Berry and Green Tea

120ml (4 fl.oz) orange juice
120ml (4 fl.oz) green tea
112g (4 oz) frozen mixed berries
1 small banana
Handful of fresh spinach

159 calories

Pour orange juice and green tea into blender
Add mixed berries
Slice and add banana
Put in spinach
Blend until smooth

*Green tea has many health benefits one of which is,
reportedly, preventing hair loss*

Fruity Treat

56g (2oz) strawberries
112g (4oz) fresh or canned pineapple
150ml (5 fl.oz) orange juice
Crushed ice

161 calories

Put strawberries into blender
Add pineapple, cut into chunks if necessary
Pour in orange juice
Whizz thoroughly in blender
Pour into glass over crushed ice

A good dose of vitamin C in this serving

Berrylumptious

120ml (4 fl.oz) skimmed milk
56g (2 oz) frozen mixed berries
180ml (6 fl.oz) orange juice

162 calories

Pour milk into blender
Add mixed berries
Pour in orange juice
Blend completely

*Berries contain antioxidants to fight the free
radicals in our bodies which cause ageing and
affect our health adversely*

Banalmondilla

240ml (8 fl.oz) skimmed milk
1 small banana
¼ teaspoon vanilla essence
Couple of drops almond extract
Pinch ground cinnamon

162 calories

Pour milk into blender
Slice and add banana
Add vanilla essence and almond extract
Blend and serve sprinkled with cinnamon

Skimmed milk is kind to your waistline

Ginger Perk

60ml (2 fl.oz) pineapple juice
120ml (4 fl.oz) orange juice
1 small banana
½ teaspoon grated ginger root
Ice cubes

167 calories

Pour pineapple juice and orange juice into
blender
Chop and add banana
Put in grated ginger and ice cubes
Blend on high setting

*Among its many medicinal properties ginger is
known for its antifungal, antibacterial and antiviral
benefits. Has to be good for you then!*

Tastebud Tantaliser

168g (6 oz) honeydew melon
4 tablespoons fat-free lemon yogurt
84g (3 oz) seedless green grapes
2 teaspoons fresh mint
Crushed ice

169 calories

Dice melon and put into blender
Spoon in yoghurt
Add grapes
Chop and add mint
Whizz until smooth and pour onto crushed
ice
Stir well and serve

*Pterostilbene, which is found in green grapes is
thought to help prevent cancer and also lower
cholesterol levels in the body. It is, however, rather
hard to pronounce!*

Carrotty Orange

2 medium sized carrots
240ml (8fl.oz) orange juice with bits
Ice

170 calories

Peel and chop carrots and put into blender
Add orange juice
Blend on high setting until smooth
Add ice and blend again

*Loads of vitamin C in one glass. This vitamin is an
antioxidant that helps us to keep healthy and
prevents damage to the cells in our bodies*

Melon Refresher

168g (6 oz) cantaloupe melon
84g (3 oz) honeydew melon
84g (3 oz) watermelon
60ml (2 fl.oz) mango juice
1 teaspoon lime juice
1 teaspoons honey
5 fresh mint leaves
Ice cubes

170 calories

Dice cantaloupe and honeydew melon
Deseed and dice watermelon
Put all melon chunks into blender
Pour in mango and lime juices
Add honey, mint leaves and ice cubes
Blend until completely smooth

*You can freeze puréed watermelon in ice cube trays
to chill drinks and add a subtle touch of flavour*

Pineapple Pick-Me Up

112g (4oz) canned pineapple
56g (2oz) strawberries
150ml (5 fl.oz) pineapple juice
Ice

171 calories

If using pineapple rings, cut into chunks and
place in blender
Add strawberries
Pour in pineapple juice
Blend thoroughly

*The nutrients in this cooling drink provide you with
natural energy*

Berrinilla

120ml (4 fl.oz) fat-free vanilla yogurt
60ml (2 fl.oz) skimmed milk
84g (3 oz) frozen cherries
84g (3 oz) frozen raspberries
Couple of drops vanilla extract
60ml (2 fl.oz) water

172 calories

Put yoghurt into blender
Pour in milk
Add fruit
Drop in vanilla extract
Add water
Blend on high setting until smooth

The humble raspberry has a high level of antioxidants which prevent deterioration of your eyes

Purple Sunset

4 tablespoons low fat vanilla yogurt
1 small peach or 112g (4 oz) frozen peach
slices
1 small banana
56g (2 oz) blueberries

172 calories

Put yoghurt into blender
Slice peach and add to blender
Chop banana and add
Put in blueberries
Whizz until smooth

*Research suggests that the chlorogenic acid in
blueberries helps to lower blood sugar levels*

Creamy Fruit Teaser

3 tablespoons low fat natural yoghurt
112g (4 oz) pineapple chunks
42g (1½ oz) frozen peach slices
56g (2 oz) blueberries
60ml (2 fl.oz) pineapple juice

175 calories

Spoon yoghurt into blender
Put in pineapple chunks
Add peach slices
Add blueberries
Pour in pineapple juice
Blend until creamy and smooth

*Plenty of health-giving antioxidants in these
blueberries*

Spicy Pumpkin

7 tablespoons pumpkin puree
120ml (4 fl.oz) water
120ml (4 fl.oz) skimmed milk
1 tablespoon clear honey
pinch of ground nutmeg
Ice

175 calories

Spoon puree into blender
Pour in water and milk
Add honey, nutmeg and ice
Blend briefly until smooth

Zinc and alphahydroxy-acids in pumpkins are
thought to help reduce signs of aging

Smooth Slimmer

1 small banana
120ml (4 fl.oz) orange juice
120ml (4fl.oz) skimmed milk

176 calories

Slice banana and put into blender
Pour in orange juice and skimmed milk
Blend thoroughly

*Bananas contain important amino acids that our
bodies need*

Green Tonic

½ avocado
Juice of 1 lime
Handful baby spinach
240ml (8 fl.oz) water

176 calories

Pour water into blender
Scoop flesh from avocado and add carefully
to water (to avoid splashing)
Squeeze lime and add juice to blender
Put in spinach
Combine until smooth

Spinach is rich in iron and helps prevent anaemia

Ripe and Rosy Rollover

60ml (2 fl.oz) vanilla yoghurt
56g (2 oz) fresh ripe rhubarb
1 small banana
120 ml (4 fl.oz) cranberry juice

176 calories

Spoon yoghurt into blender
Chop and add rhubarb
Slice and add banana
Pour in cranberry juice
Whizz well until smooth

Cranberry is great for the kidneys and urinary tract

Berry and Citrus

56g (2 oz) blueberries
120ml (4 fl.oz) orange juice
½ tangerine
½ orange
½ grapefruit
Ice cubes

177 calories

Put blueberries into blender
Pour in orange juice
Add segments of citrus fruits
Pop in ice cubes
Whizz until smooth

Low in calories but high in vitamins, grapefruit is an ideal weight loss fruit. Some people, though, are on medications like statins, that clash with it. If you are one of those, use 1½ tangerines instead to keep the calorie count for this smoothie

Peachy Mango Temptation

112g (4 oz) frozen peach slices
112g (4 oz) frozen mango chunks
120ml (4 fl.oz) peach nectar
1 tablespoon lime juice

184 calories

Place peach slices in blender
Add mango chunks
Pour in peach nectar
Add lime juice
Whizz in blender until smooth

Peaches are low in calories with lots of healthy minerals and vitamins

Merry Berry Cherry

120ml (4 fl.oz) fat-free natural yoghurt
112g (4 oz) strawberries
112g (4 oz) frozen cherries
2 tsp. ground flax seed
¾ tsp. pure vanilla extract

185 calories

Spoon yoghurt into blender
Halve and add strawberries
Put in cherries
Add flax seed and vanilla extract
Blend on high setting

*Cherries contain anthocyanins: natural pigments
said to help to prevent cancer. Cherries taste good
too!*

Raspberry and Peach Delight

112g (4 oz) peach yoghurt
112g (4 oz) frozen raspberries
180 ml (6 fl.oz) orange juice

188 calories

Spoon yoghurt into blender
Add raspberries
Pour in orange juice
Blend thoroughly

Raspberries are very good for cleansing your gut!

Lemony Apricot & Mango

180ml (6 fl.oz) skimmed milk
3 apricots
112g (4 oz) frozen mango slices
2 tablespoons lemon juice
¼ teaspoon vanilla essence
Ice cubes

193 calories

Pour milk into blender
Slice apricots
Add apricots to blender
Add in mango slices
Pour in lemon juice, vanilla essence and ice cubes
Blend until smooth and creamy

Apricots, whilst low in calories, are high in dietary fibre, vitamins and minerals

Spicy Almond with Kale

1 small banana
56g (2 oz) kale, stems removed
180ml (6 fl.oz) almond milk
¾ tablespoon almond butter
pinch each of ground cinnamon, nutmeg and
ginger.

194 calories

Slice banana before placing in blender
Chop and add kale
Pour in almond milk
Add almond butter
Put in spices
Blend until completely smooth

*Almond milk is thought to help reduce the risk of
Alzheimers and osteoporosis, because it contains
lots of vitamin D which helps in cell building*

Fruity Oaty Shake

180ml (6 fl.oz) fat-free natural yoghurt
112g (4 oz) frozen raspberries
60ml (2 fl.oz) skimmed milk
1 tablespoon oatmeal
60ml (2 fl.oz) water

196 calories

Spoon yoghurt into blender
Add raspberries
Pour in milk
Add oatmeal
Pour in water
Blend everything thoroughly

Oats are an excellent source of many healthy nutrients, two of which are magnesium and protein. Magnesium is said to combat stress and protein is essential for energy and to rebuild tissue body tissue

Tasty Tummy Soother

120ml (4 fl.oz) fat-free natural yoghurt
56g (2oz) papaya
56g (2oz) frozen sliced peaches
1 small pear
1 teaspoon ground flax seed
½ tsp ground ginger
2 mint leaves

204 calories

Spoon yoghurt into blender
Peel, deseed and cube papaya
Add peaches and papaya to yoghurt
Peel, chop and add pear
Put in flax seed and ginger
Blend thoroughly and garnish with mint
leaves

*Among its many health benefits papaya relieves
digestion problems, improves your skin and protects
your heart and eyes*

Peanut Butter Creamer

4 tablespoons fat-free vanilla yogurt
120ml (4 fl.oz) pineapple juice
1 tablespoon of smooth peanut butter
120ml (4 fl.oz) almond milk
Ice

206 calories

Spoon yoghurt into blender
Pour in pineapple juice
Add peanut butter
Pour in almond milk
Pop in ice
Blend thoroughly

Americans eat enough peanut butter each year to cover the floor of the Grand Canyon, but there's still enough left for your smoothie wherever you live!

Blueberry Orange

4 tablespoons fat-free vanilla yoghurt
112g (4oz) blueberries
120ml (4 fl.oz) orange juice
120ml (4 fl.oz) skimmed milk
½ teaspoon vanilla essence

206 calories

Spoon yoghurt into blender
Add blueberries
Pour in orange juice and milk
Add vanilla essence
Blend until completely smooth

*With superstar blueberries, vitamin C rich orange
juice and bone-healthy calcium in the milk, it's a
truly health-giving drink*

Spicy Nutty Pear, Orange and Rocket

120ml (4 fl.oz) natural fat-free yogurt
1 teaspoon of ground ginger
1small ripe pear
1 tablespoon chopped walnuts
84g (3 oz) rocket (arugula)
120ml (4 fl.oz) almond milk
Ice cubes

211 calories

Spoon yoghurt into blender
Add ginger
Core, chop and add pear
Add walnuts and rocket
Pour in almond milk
Pop in ice cubes
Blend completely

*Walnuts contain vitamins, minerals and
antioxidants and also help to give you energy*

Pear, Peach and Strawberry

4 tablespoons fat-free natural yoghurt
1 small soft pear
1 small ripe peach
112g (4oz) strawberries
120ml (4 fl.oz) coconut water

216 calories

Spoon yoghurt into blender
Peel and slice pear and peach before adding
to blender
Halve and add strawberries
Pour in coconut water
Whizz on high setting until well combined

*For a mild laxative look no further than pears. It's
the pectin in them that has this effect on the body*

Grapefully Smoothful

112g (4 oz) green seedless grapes
120ml (4 fl.oz) grape juice
84g (3 oz) frozen blueberries
75 ml (2½ fl.oz) almond milk

217 calories

Put grapes into blender
Pour in grape juice
Add blueberries
Pour in almond milk
Whizz thoroughly

Grapes are good for the heart. They raise nitric oxide levels in the blood which helps to prevent blood clots and staves off heart attacks and strokes

Strawberry-Kiwi Fantasia

210ml (7 fl.oz) apple juice
1 small banana
1 kiwi fruit
56g (2 oz) frozen strawberries

223 calories

Pour apple juice into blender
Chop and add banana
Halve kiwi fruit, scoop out flesh and put in
blender
Add strawberries
Blend thoroughly

*Give your immune system a helping hand with all
this vitamin C*

Pomegranate surprise

1 small banana
1 kiwi fruit
70g (2½ oz) blueberries
56g (2 oz) strawberries
90ml (3 fl.oz) pomegranate juice

224 calories

Slice banana and put into blender
Halve kiwi and scoop flesh into blender
Add blueberries
Halve strawberries and add
Pour in pomegranate juice
Whizz until smooth

Pomegranate juice is a tasty way to settle stomach upsets

Berry Beetroot

4 tablespoons fat-free natural yoghurt
168g (6 oz) blueberries
84g (3 oz) frozen raspberries
56g (2 oz) cooked beetroot
60ml (2 fl.oz) orange juice
Stevia

227 calories

Spoon yoghurt into blender
Put in blueberries
Add raspberries
Peel, slice and add beetroot
Pour in orange juice
Add stevia if sweeter taste is required
Blend everything

The beta cyanin in beetroot helps detoxify your liver

Blueberry and Bananalicous

150ml (5 fl oz) apple juice
120ml (4 fl.oz) natural yoghurt
1 small banana
112g (4oz) blueberries

229 calories

Pour apple juice into blender
Spoon in yoghurt
Chop and add banana
Put in blueberries
Combine until smooth

*There is exciting new research suggesting that
regular consumption of blueberries may not only be
beneficial for improving memory but might also
slow down, or postpone, various cognitive problems
associated with aging*

Berrylicious Banana

60ml (2 fl.oz) soya milk
1 small ripe banana
1 tablespoon smooth peanut butter
168g (6 oz) raspberries
Crushed ice

230 calories

Pour soya milk into blender
Slice and add banana
Put in peanut butter
Add raspberries and ice
Blend to a smooth consistency

Peanut butter contains resveratrol -an antioxidant which, it is thought, helps prevent heart disease and cancer

Smoothberry and Beetroot

1 teaspoon honey
60ml (2 fl.oz) low-fat natural yoghurt
112g (4 oz) raw beetroot
2 tablespoons granola
168g (6 oz) mixed blueberries
120ml (4 fl.oz) freshly squeezed orange
juice
Ice cubes

230 calories

Spoon honey and yoghurt into blender
Peel, finely chop and add beetroot
Add granola and blueberries
Pour in orange juice
Pop in ice
Blend on high setting until completely
smooth

*Betaine in beetroot may help to cheer you up
because it increases serotonin, a mood enhancer
which is naturally produced in the body*

Minty Avocado, Lime and Mango

½ small avocado
168g (6 oz) frozen mango slices
1 tablespoon lime juice
1 tablespoon chopped fresh mint
Stevia
240ml (8 fl.oz) water

234 calories

Scoop flesh of avocado into blender
Add mango slices
Pour in lime juice
Add chopped mint
Put in stevia to taste
Pour in water
Blend thoroughly

*The avocado is believed to have originated in
Mexico, where the name comes from an Aztec word:
'ahuacatl' meaning 'testicle' which refers to the
fruit's shape (just thought you'd like to know that!)*

Pear, Peach and Cinnamon

120ml (4 fl.oz) apple juice
120ml (4 fl.oz) fat-free natural yoghurt
1 small ripe pear
84g (3 oz) frozen peach slices
½ teaspoon cinnamon

238 calories

Pour apple juice into blender
Spoon in yoghurt
Core, chop and add pear
Add peach slices
Sprinkle with cinnamon
Whizz until completely combined

*Pears boost your immune system, help prevent
osteoporosis, increase energy and aid your
digestion – in short, they're very good for you!*

Mildly Nutty and Fruity

1 tablespoon ground flax seed
4 tablespoons fat-free natural yoghurt.
120ml (4 fl.oz) pineapple juice
1 kiwi fruit
½ papaya
84g (3 oz) frozen mango slices

246 calories

Put flax seed and yoghurt into blender
Pour in pineapple juice
Halve kiwi fruit, scoop out flesh and add
Deseed, peel, chop and add papaya
Add mango slices
Blitz until smooth

*Low in calories, ground flaxseed provides you with
essential vitamins and minerals in this delicious
smoothie*

Calorifically Speaking...

The following chart will help you in several ways:

- If you want to vary any of the recipes you can check your calorie count and balance each smoothie to fit in with your day's allowance
- If you decide to become adventurous and invent your own smoothies, you can use the chart to help plan your ingredients and your calorie intake
- It will help you become familiar with the calorie counts of a wide variety of foods

It is arranged in alphabetical order for ease of use and gives the calories (kcal) for the various measuring units used in the recipes in this book.

Whole fruit and vegetables, being natural and therefore variable in size can be difficult to "pin down" in precise amounts of calories. Where these are listed please regard this as referring to a medium size item unless otherwise stated.

Ingredient	1 item	28g (1 oz)	30ml (1 fl.oz)	1 Teaspoon	1 Tablespoon
Almond butter		177		34	101
Almond extract				11	
Almond milk, unsweetened			3		
Apple	80	15			
Apple juice			15		
Apricots, canned		14			
Apricots, fresh	17				
Avocado	322	50			
Banana, medium	105	25			
Banana, small	72	25			
Banana, v. small (under 6in.)	55	25			
Beet leaves	7	8			
Beetroot, cooked		12			
Beetroot, raw		12			

Ingredient	1 item	28g (1 oz)	30ml (1 fl.oz)	1 Teaspoon	1 Tablespoon
Berries , mixed		14			
Blackberries		12			
Blueberries		16			
Broccoli		9			
Carrot	25	12			
Carrot juice			12		
Cayenne pepper				6	
Celery stalk	6	4			
Cherries, frozen		13			
Cinnamon, ground				6	
Cloves, ground				6	
Cocoa powder, unsweetened				4	12
Coconut water			6		
Coffee, brewed			1		
Coffee, instant granules				2	

Ingredient	1 item	28g (1 oz)	30ml (1 fl.oz)	1 Teaspoon	1 Tablespoon
Cranberries		13			
Cranberry juice			15		
Cucumber, peeled	24	3			
Flax seed, ground				12	36
Ginger, ground				6	18
Ginger, root		22		2	
Granola		95			35
Grapefruit	72				
Grape Juice			21		
Grapes		20			
Green tea			0		
Honey				20	60
Ice		0			
Kale leaves		14			
Kiwi fruit	29	13			
Lemon without peel	17				

Ingredient	1 item	28g (1 oz)	30ml (1 fl.oz)	1 Teaspoon	1 Tablespoon
Lemon juice			7		4
Lemon zest				1	
Lime juice	10		8	1	4
Mango juice			15		
Mango pieces, frozen		17			
Matcha				6	
Melon, cantaloupe		10			
Melon, honeydew		10			
Milk, skimmed			11		
Mint, fresh					1
Nectarine	60				
Nutmeg, ground				12	36
Oatmeal					18
Onion				1	4
Orange	62				
Orange, large	86				

Ingredient	1 item	28g (1 oz)	30ml (1 fl.oz)	1 Teaspoon	1 Tablespoon
Orange juice			15		
Papaya, small	59	11			
Parsley		10			1
Passion fruit	17				
Peach nectar		17			
Peach slices, frozen		11			
Peach, fresh	55				
Peanut butter, smooth					94
Pear	96				
Pear, small	80				
Pepper, ground				5	
Pineapple juice			17		
Pineapple, canned		17			
Pineapple, fresh		14			
Pomegranate juice			17		
Prune juice			22		

Ingredient	1 item	28g (1 oz)	30ml (1 fl.oz)	1 Teaspoon	1 Tablespoon
Pumpkin puree		10			10
Raspberries		15			
Rhubarb pieces		6			
Rhubarb stalk	11				
Rice milk			15		
Rocket		4			
Salt		0		0	
Sorbet, orange		25			
Soya milk, unsweetened			8		
Soya milk, vanilla			14		
Spinach		7			
Strawberries		9			
Stevia		0		0	0
Tabasco sauce				1	
Tangerine	36				

Ingredient	1 item	28g (1 oz)	30ml (1 fl.oz)	1 Teaspoon	1 Tablespoon
Tomato	22	5			
Tomato, small	18	5			
Tomato juice		5			
Vanilla essence				2	
Vanilla extract				12	
Walnuts		194			40
Water		0		0	0
Watercress		4			
Watermelon		9			
Yoghurt, lemon, fat-free		24			12
Yoghurt, natural, fat-free		16			8
Yoghurt, peach, fat-free		17			8
Yoghurt, vanilla, fat-free		16			8

Index of Smoothies

Smoothies are listed in order of calorie content, both in the index below and throughout the book. You may like to use a highlighter to mark ones you particularly enjoy so that you can easily find them again.

151-200 Calories

201-246 Calories

Printed in Great Britain
by Amazon.co.uk, Ltd.,
Marston Gate.